Curing Constipation Naturally

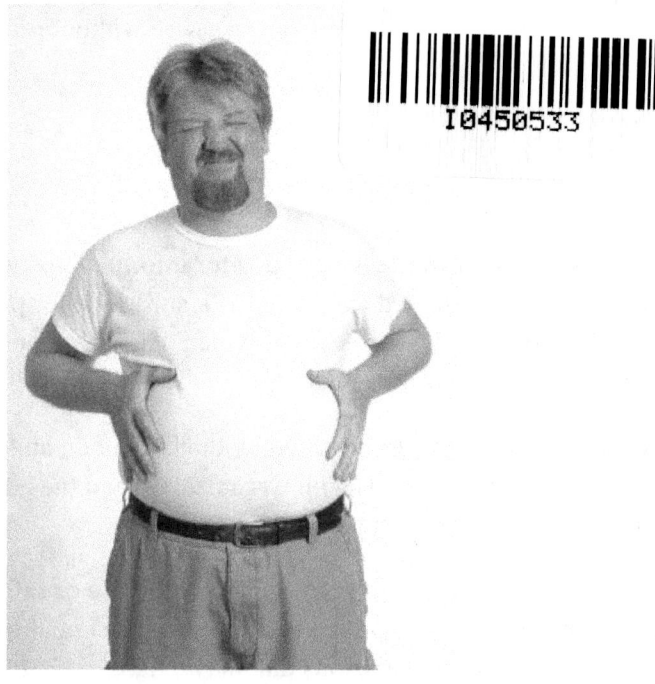

Health Learning Series

By Dueep J. Singh

Mendon Cottage Books

JD-Biz Publishing

Check out some of the other Healthy Gardening Series books at Amazon.com

Gardening Series on Amazon

Check out some of the other Health Learning Series books at Amazon.com

Health Learning Series on Amazon

Table of Contents

Introduction

Did you know that more than 7.4 million people in the United States alone suffer from some form of constipation? Multiply that about 10 times or more and you are going to get the global statistics for this tiresome digestive problem. This means about 12% of the world population suffers from chronic or mild dyschezia – which is the medical term for costiveness or constipation. USD260 million are spent every year by people looking for over the counter remedies, and around USD7 billion is being spent on healthcare for just this one particular digestive problem, in the United States alone.

What Is Constipation?

Have you found yourself suffering from irregular bowel movements, especially when you need to empty out your digestive system of fecal solids just two or three times a week? Are these stools hard and do you find it difficult to eliminate them? You are suffering from constipation.

Constipation has been the bane of human beings for millenniums. The major factors causing this sort of infrequent bowel movements include change of diet, which means that you are not drinking enough water, or you are not eating food which is rich in fiber. Also, living a sedentary lifestyle and not indulging much in exercise or physical activity can cause constipation.

Constipation can also because as a side effect, when you take a number of drugs. People suffering from hypothyroidism are also going to suffer from occasional constipation.

Are there any medical reasons for this ailment? It is not caused by bacteria and viruses. However, scientific studies say that women are more vulnerable to this problem than are men. Dieting can also cause constipation because you are not eating those essential nutrients which are needed by your body to keep your system healthy and ""moving regularly."

Drugs can also be a major cause of constipation with this problem as a side effect. So if you are taking antacids, antispasmodics, diuretics, antihistamines and painkillers in large quantities, you are going to fall a prey to this problem sometime or the other in the near future.

Symptoms of Constipation

Thanks to the discomfort of not having voided your alimentary canal, you may find yourself suffering from lethargy, headaches, tension, pain in your stomach, distention and even bloating. If you manage to get to the bathroom, these tools are going to be hard and you may have this feeling of "emptying" being incomplete.

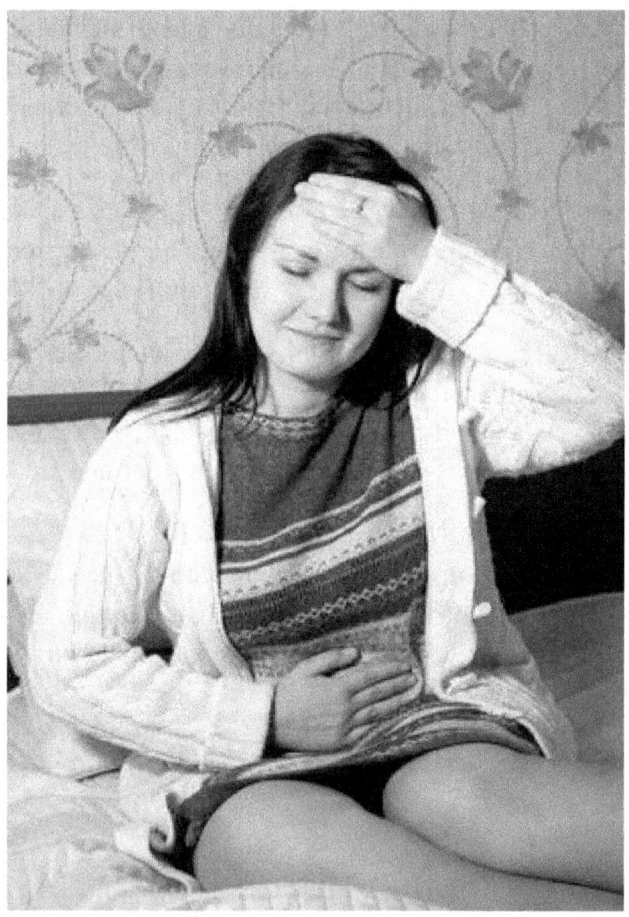

Rules to Prevent Constipation

Prevention is much better than cure, when you are faced with this ailment. If you digestive system is weak, you may want to start hearing it by drinking fresh fruit juice diluted in water. This is easy to digest and gets your system moving. It is much better to eat fruit on an empty stomach. This fruit diet was one of the most common practices used by the ancients to get rid of and cure a large number of diseases.

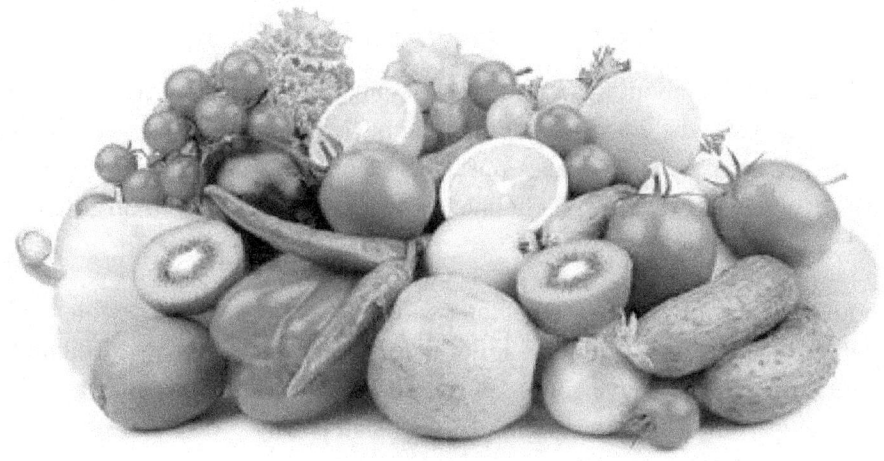

Fruit juice therapy is basically a long-term process, and it takes a long time for you to heal your system. But as they are healthy items to take regularly, you can drink fresh fruit juice in the morning and in the afternoon.

Drink about 16 ounces of juice every day. The fruit and vegetables should be seasonal. Do not add sugar or honey to this fruit juice. That is because our body is capable of producing sugar through the food being eaten on its own, naturally.

Eating Skins

The first time I saw a woman eating up an orange without peeling it was sitting in a bus in Piccadilly Circus in London. I was astonished, when I saw her just speak out a nice juicy orange from her bag and sink her strong teeth into it, peel included. I had seen people eating apples without peeling, but this was quite something else.

My surprise was because since childhood, I had been taught to peel fruit and vegetables before I ate them. But here was a fellow passenger, crunching away on an orange, – I hope she had washed it beforehand, to get rid of the pesticides and dirt-and thus gaining all the benefits of its orange peel.

Now the good thing about this was that her stomach would be completely free of parasites, thanks to the citric oil found in the peel. The only worry was, she was adding to her toxin intake, because unless those oranges were organically grown, she was eating peel drenched in chemicals, pesticides and other toxin filled agricultural products.

So should you eat any fruit or vegetable, which you have peeled previously? Yes, you can, if the skin is not tough or solid. Skins of organically grown fruit and vegetables are going to have a number of nutrients and minerals. They are also going to keep your digestive system healthy. That is why, I do not peel cucumbers, scrape potato skins, peel off Apple skins and so on, when I am feeling hungry. Just wash them properly, and eat along with skin.

A dietitian friend told me that the best way in which one could keep her digestive system moving properly was to drink half a glass of water before eating a meal. That gave the stomach a liquid base in which the masticated solids could be mixed easily after every meal. This was extremely helpful in the digestion and the assimilation of foodstuffs.

Harmful Effects of Constipation

Constipation is the forerunner to a number of diseases. That is because the food which has not been excreted and eliminated in the regular manner is going to rot in our digestive system. It is going to create toxic wastes in the form of gas and poisons. All these toxic wastes and poisons are going to mix up in the blood and reach the rest of the body through the circulatory system.

This is going to weaken the body. It is also going to make the body more vulnerable to infections because the resistance of the body has lessened, due to this toxic poisoning. You are going to feel lethargic, your stomach is going to feel bloated and you are going to find difficulty in breathing.

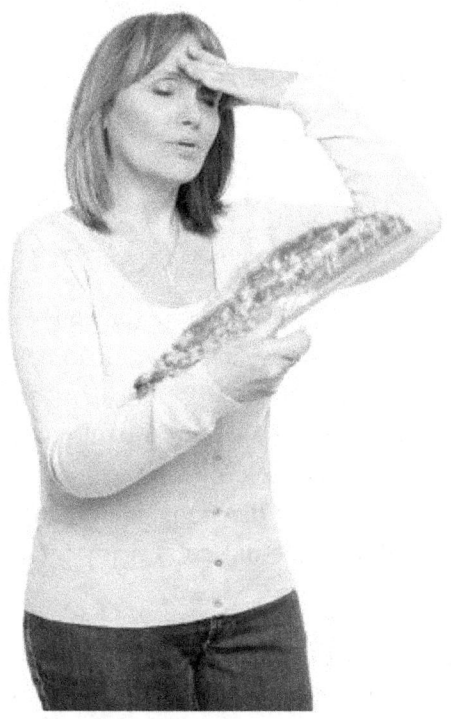

Constipation also creates halitosis, because those toxic wastes are being removed through any opening, including your air passage through your mouth. You may also feel feverish, nauseated and fall prey to headaches.

A chronic case of constipation can give rise to piles and also sciatica.

Easy Tips for Controlling Constipation

Constipation in itself is not an ailment but it is the sum total of your daily mental and physical activities, diet, and inactivity too. Never try using any sort of medicine, which causes diarrhea in order to get rid of constipation. There was a time when giving soap and salt enemas to all the members of the family every morning in order to get their systems moving was considered fashionable. Every quack and Barber recommended it, when they were not bleeding their patients with lancets and leeches.

That is definitely a quack remedy because it only weakens the system.

In the same way, do not feed your child with castor oil in milk, thinking that you are going to cure a case of constipation. Then the child has not been given enough of liquid or enough of fibrous diet in order to get his system, moving naturally, you are ruining his natural digestive system with the use of castor oil, and such other emetics.

Start eating more raw fruit and vegetables. Try going to the bathroom more often, even though you do not want to empty out your bowels. That activity done at a particular time regularly is going to regularize your system.

Many people suffer from constipation because they have not eaten enough of food in order to produce enough of waste materials to be eliminated. Remember that the waste materials are going to solidify into small chunks of solids after all the liquid intake has been assimilated and absorbed by the body. If there are not enough of fibrous materials in the diet you take, you are going to find yourself suffering from constipation because the stomach did not have enough of fiber to bind all that waste material together and get it ready for elimination.

You need to rest after you have eaten a meal. We have this unfortunate tendency to have lunch and then get back to work as soon as possible, because we are watching the clock. We do not have time to relax and allow our body to rest a little, for at least half an hour after we have had a meal. This naturally has an adverse effect on our digestive systems.

Mankind has been geared by Mother Nature to digest its food in a leisurely fashion. However, in the 21st century, that is not the option for a number of us. So back we go back to our sedentary lifestyle, sitting crouched up in front of our computers or on our desks, not giving our stomachs the opportunity to digest the food in a proper manner.

Actually, the ancients suggested that you needed to walk about 100 steps after you had your meals. That was to set the digestive system going and activate all the stomach muscles. How many of us do this? I asked my friends and acquaintances if they did that taking a walk – exercise after having a meal. All of them told me that they hated exercising! And especially not after a meal. Just getting back to their desks was their top priority even if they felt sleepy throughout the afternoon.

No wonder we are suffering from constipation, one and all.

Diet

So here are the diet items of the ancients, who lived 900 years like Methuselah. He ate lentils, especially those with their skins on. He also drank plenty of fresh milk and ate butter and milk products in abundance. But that last is something we are not going to do, because we do not spend the whole day in shepherding activities, or doing other sorts of hard physical labor, which burns up all that butter and fatty milk products.

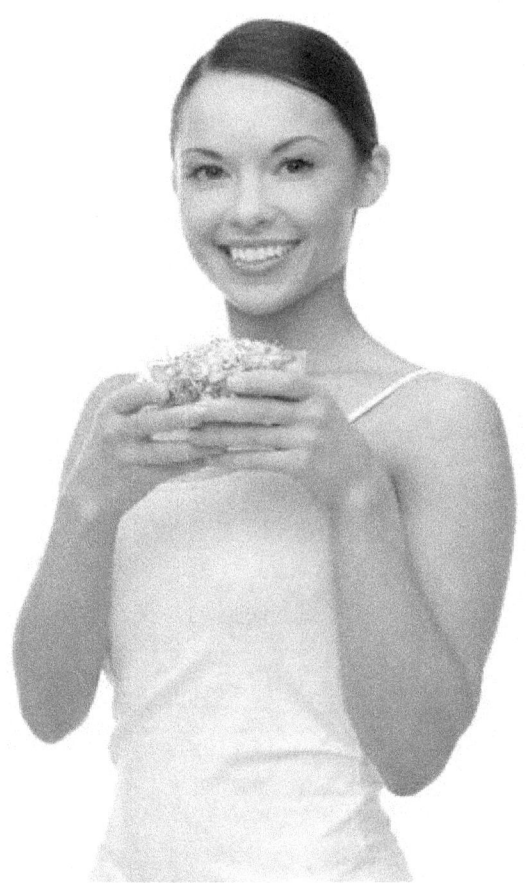

We need to eat sprouted lentils and cereals like sprouted wheat, sprouted Mung, sprouted white gram – which incidentally was fed to horses in order to increase their strength and give them lots of energy – boiled vegetables, green leafy vegetables, salads and other vegetable-based food items in our daily diet.

Spinach juice, orange juice, lemons, turnips, apples, figs, cabbage, papaya, guavas , and other fruit are good fiber producing food items.

Other fiber producing items include porridge, freshly ground wheat, which has not been refined and has the wheat bran still included, and other natural cereals have to be eaten every day. You need to eat at least 450 g of these cereals, every day in some form or the other.

The only problem is that we eat breads made of refined flour. Consider that to be a glutinous mass which is going to encourage constipation. The moment it reaches the stomach, it, not having any fiber content is just going to stick to any surface. And if there is no water content already present in your stomach, it is going to rot there and produce toxins.

You do not get fruit fiber in fruit juice. That can only be obtained by eating fresh fruit.

I remember an acquaintance who used to eat a constipation laxative made up of husks and cereal bran, regularly with her breakfast. She was very happy in the initial stages, because according to her our system got cleared, thanks to the emetic properties of that wheat bran/husks mixture.

A couple of weeks later, she told me that that laxative was useless and ineffective. What had happened? The normal digestive process had been disturbed with the use of this natural remedy. The system had begun relying on this powder in order to activate itself. So the body soon reached the stage when it had begun relying on artificial methods in order to get it working, instead of the normal digestive process.

This is something all those people selling you over the counter laxative remedies are definitely not going to tell you. That is why you shell out about USD260 million every year – believe it or not – on over the counter laxatives, which are going to work in the initial stages but are going to get ineffective in just a couple of weeks.

So my suggestion is, prevent constipation from happening by changing your lifestyle and changing your diet immediately.

Beans

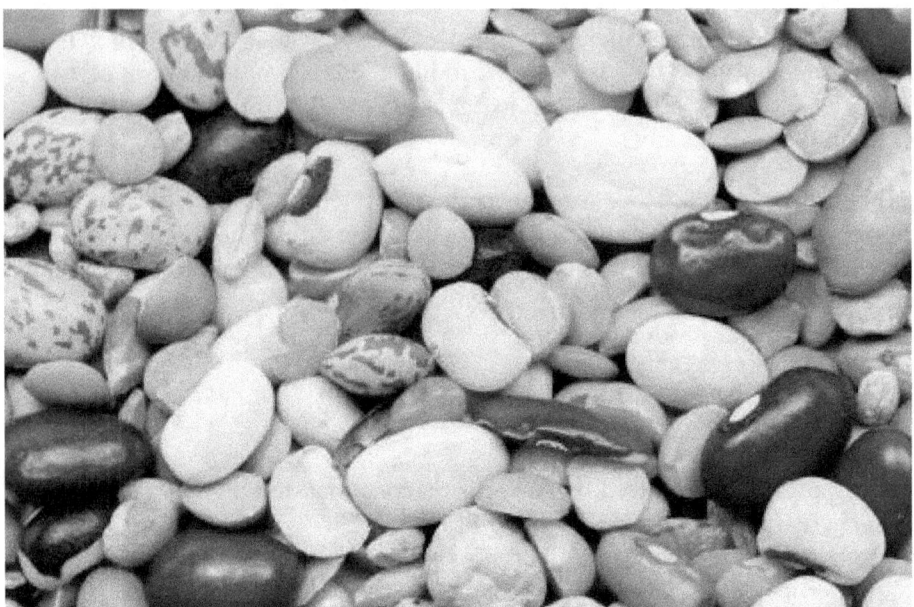

Beans are among the best available vegetarian protein source in the world. They are also important food components of every existing diet in the world. Beans, being a mixture of carbohydrates and proteins may be difficult to digest. However, this is good because a diet of beans makes you feel less hungry.

Also, your digestive system is never going to suffer from constipation, thanks to the rich fiber content in beans. Choose plain beans and cook them at home. Avoid refried, fatty, processed and baked tinned beans. These items are disastrous for any weight loss routine. That is because they have more calories and carbohydrates in them.

Sweet Almond Oil

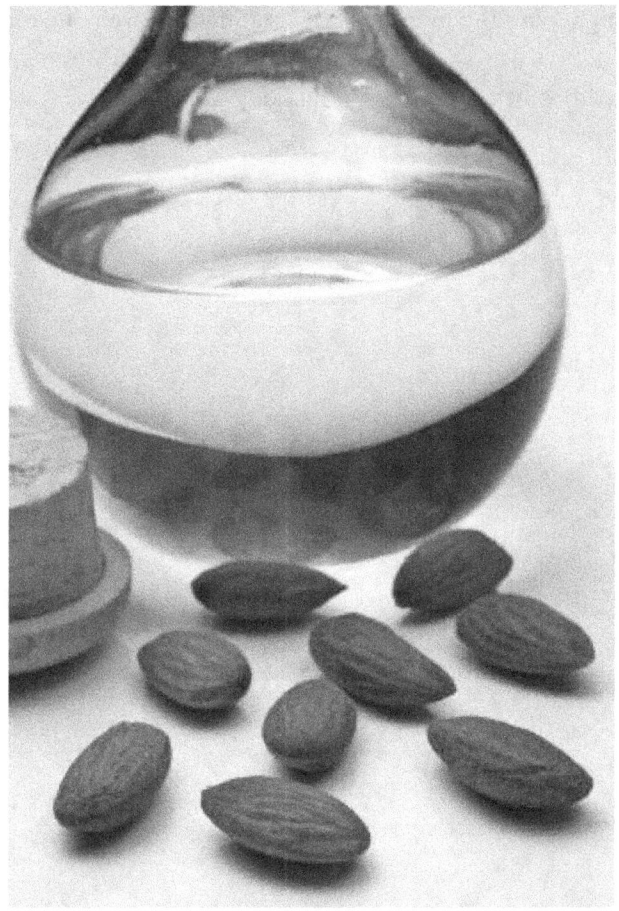

Sweet almond oil is rather expensive because it is so much in demand as a skin moisturizer and beautifier. But in the East, it has been used as a natural remedy for curing constipation for millenniums. People put two drops of sweet almond oil in the glassful of milk they drink for breakfast. No worries about tummy problems or constipation ever.

I remember I buying a bottle of sweet almond oil from my friendly neighborhood grocers'. And I received a funny sort of look from him, when he asked me genially whether I wanted it to cure constipation, because if that was the main reason, he could give me a smaller [and thus more expensive] bottle. But I told him that I wanted it for my skin. Voila, the funny look!

Sweet almond oil is used in many parts of the East on the forehead and scalp supposedly in order to "cool" your head, enhance your brain power and intellectual strength, and the mere idea of wasting this precious oil as a skin moisturizer and lotion was shocking and anathema to him! I am sure he started to consider me a faddy sort of snob, from that day on!

Honey

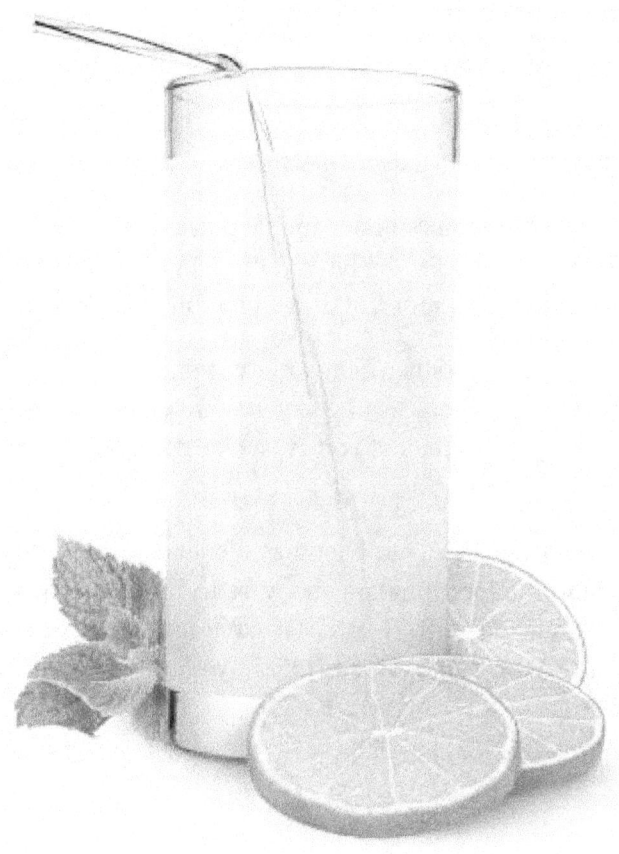

Lime juice with honey is excellent for you.

Did you know that honey is the best way in which you can cure constipation? Even people who have been suffering from chronic constipation, which has been ailing them for a number of years, can heal themselves by eating one teaspoonful of honey, as often as they can, with some ginger juice.

Try drinking half a teaspoonful of honey in boiled milk before you go to sleep. Also, try eating nothing solid for one full day, but drinking plenty of fresh fruit juices and water. This is going to get your system moving, because there is enough of liquid in your stomach to regularize the natural activity of your alimentary canal.

One teaspoonful of olive oil after every meal is good for you. It is also going to prevent constipation. **Tomato juice is also excellent to cure constipation.**

Remember to eat just the pulp of a tomato, when you are eating it in salad in juice form or in raw form. The seeds often cause problems in your tummy.

Wake up at Dawn. Wash your mouth out and then drink one glass of fresh water. [Waking up at Dawn is strictly for the birds for me, but the ancients did that, because they thought that not a moment of the precious day should be wasted.]

This was a rule which I found rather funny, but it is still being practiced by people in rural India. Clench your teeth when you are emptying out your bowels. Supposedly, this fixes your teeth, and you are never going to suffer from shaking teeth ever again.

I am being a little bit risqué here, but I bet they clenched their teeth automatically if they were suffering from constipation and were trying to get their system and clear of all that accumulated stuff. Even so, what is so difficult about clenching your teeth, and if it really sets the more firmly in your gums, so much the better.

Traditional Rose Jam- Gulkand

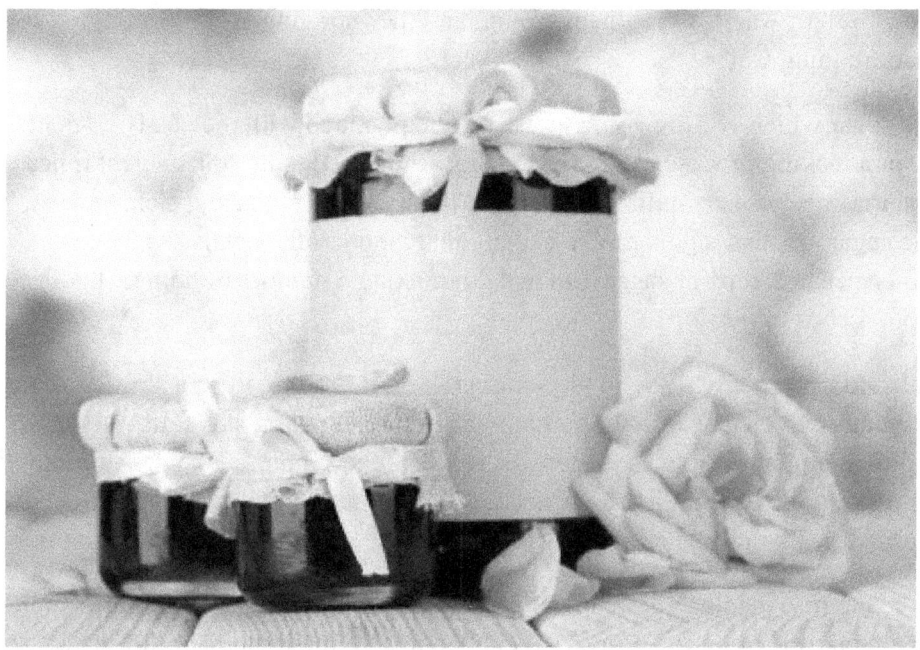

Hyperacidity is supposedly controlled with Gulkand and also, if you are suffering from constipation, you are going to find your digestive system functioning better with this Rose jam.

The best thing I like about Gulkand is that once it is made, it is going to last for years and years. One of my relatives made it with honey, but I guess that to be overkill. After all, I am putting sugar in it, am I not.

However, if you have plenty of honey around, you can make it with honey. But that is going to make it even more powerful. That means you are just going to be eating half a teaspoon, three times a day. This antioxidant is a mild laxative, and that is why it will keep your system clear and healthy.

How to collect wild rose petals – if you find red rose petals growing in the wild, how lucky you are. This is going to have more percentage of essential oils, especially if you have Rosa Damascena around. Somehow, I do not find cultivated rose hybrids to have such a great amount of required essential oils.

Make sure that the rose petals which you collect are pesticide free by washing them thoroughly. Also get rid of the insects and dust. I normally dump them in a bucket full of water, swish them around and then strain the petals through a sieve under running water.

The sugar which you are going to use can be pounded with the petals, to make the jam making process easier. That is how they used to do it in ancient times. You may also use crystallized sugar, but that is going to make it sickly sweet. The sugar amount is going to be exactly that much as the petals. So 2 cups of petals means 2 cups of sugar. But as I am making a number of bottles, I collect about 4 cups of petals.

Gulkand is normally made in the summer. And it is going to be a slow cooking of the petals and the sugar in the sun in wide mouthed glass jars. Gulkand is definitely not made in plastic utensils. It seems the Empress NoorJahan promoted the making of rose jam in Mogul aristocratic circles, but then, we already know her historically has the lady who discovered rose oil through condensation.

Place the rose petals directly in the jars, in alternate layers. Alternating with the rose petals are going to be sugar layers. Do not fill the jar to the brim. Now, cover tightly and place out in the sun. The moisture is going to cook the jam into a jammy consistency. Give the bottle a really good shake occasionally so that the jam gets a good chance to settle down well. Your long-lasting Gulkand is going to be cooked in 2 to 3 months, in the summer. Enjoy.

Mint Tea

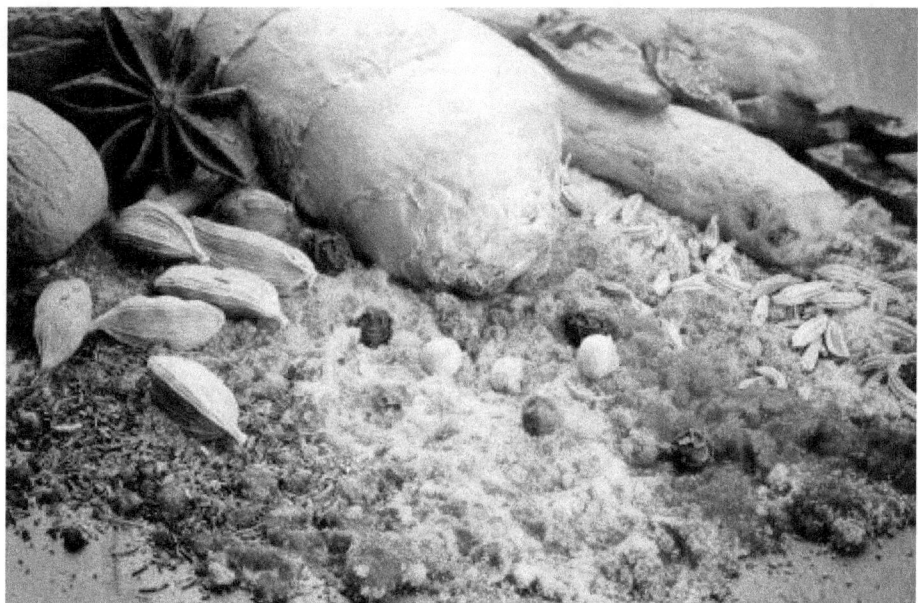

The color of the mint tea is going to depend on the time you infused it in hot water, and the number of leaves used.

Mint tea is extremely popular in the East, when the leaves are boiled, just like you would do to ordinary tea leaves. This mint tea made up of 5 to 10 leaves is normally given to teenage children, so that they have a healthy skin, and are not worried about tummy problems through eating lots of junk food.

In fact, since ancient times, when people did not know about tea, except in China and Tibet, mint leaves and basil leaves were made into hot tea infusions and drunk, twice a day, morning and evening. This was supposed to keep the whole system healthy.

Take out the juice of five – 10 mint leaves, by just grinding them with a little bit of water in a blender. A tablespoonful of this juice, taken every day in water is going to cure you of constipation.

Lovage for Stomach Related Problems

The best use, to which you can put Bishops Weed is to use it as a sovereign remedy to cure any sort of ailment, which is related to the stomach. That means this is the surefire cure for indigestion, gas problems, constipation, parasites in the stomach, tummy ache etc.

If you are suffering from gastric problems brought on due to constipation, just take one teaspoonful of Bishops Weed. Now add a little bit of rock salt. Chew it slowly and allow the saliva to mix with this mouthful. Now drink a glass of warm water or buttermilk. You are immediately going to find relief.

Carrots

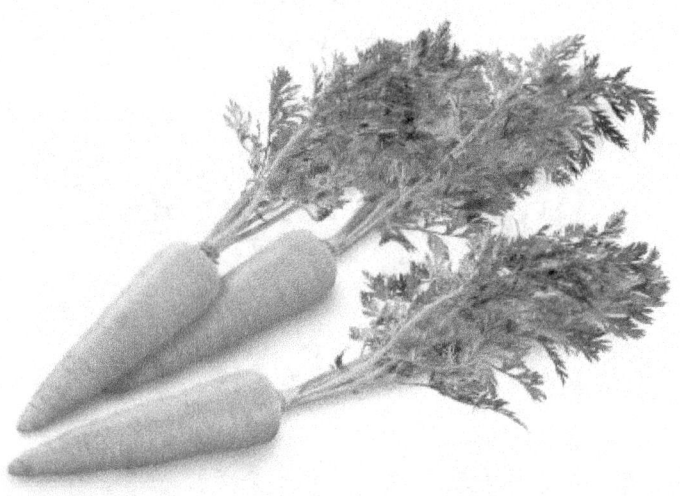

Carrot juice taken regularly every morning is going to clear up your system so that you never suffer from constipation. You may want to add one spoon of ginger juice and one spoon of lemon juice to half a cup of carrot juice.

Add a little rock salt and a little bit of roasted cumin seeds and a pinch of asafoetida to this juice mixture. Drink this morning and evening. This remedy has been used through millenniums to get rid of dyspepsia and indigestion.

If you do not want to go through the spice route, you can also try this remedy of drinking half a cup of carrot juice, and with a little bit of rock salt, first thing in the morning on an empty stomach.

Cannot find rock salt around? Okay, then drink half a cup of carrot juice with 2 teaspoons onion juice, once a day.

Try drinking 2 tablespoons of the juice of carrots leaves twice a day.

Make a chutney of two carrots, 10 g raw ginger, two cloves of garlic, one pinch of black salt, and 3 tablespoons of vinegar. This chutney is a well-known flatulence remedy.

Half a cup of carrot juice, one spoon ginger juice, 2 tablespoons lemon juice and half a teaspoonful of sacred basil juice. Mix them together and divide into two parts, each portion to be drunk in the morning and evening. Try this for three days and see if your chronic constipation problem is not cured.

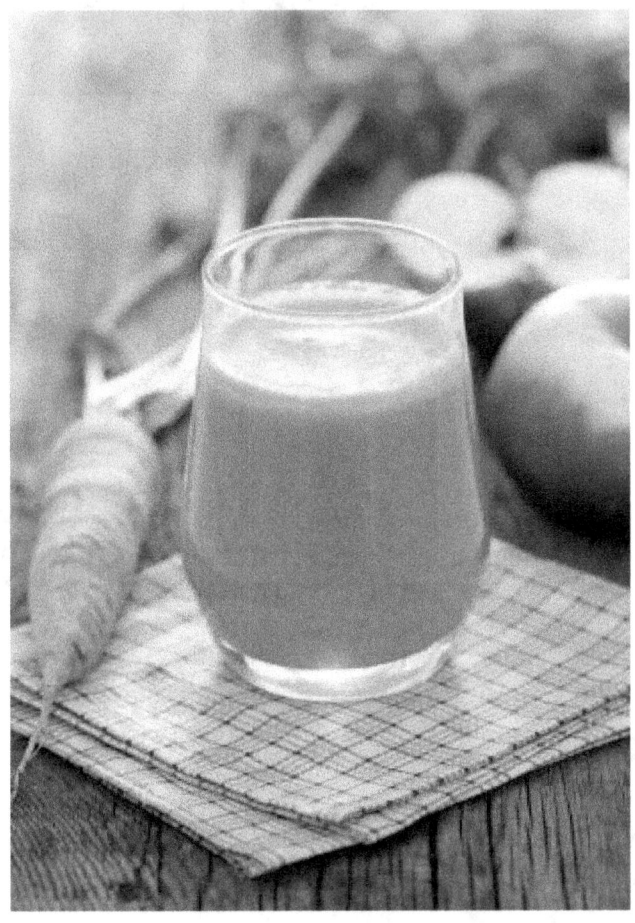

Or you can alternatively try. Hundred grams carrot juice, 150 g spinach juice, 50 g tomato juice. Mix them all up and add two teaspoons full of honey. Drink this for a few days. Try avoiding foods like bread made of self raising flour, which it does not have dietary fibers.

Try adding some boiled carrots to molasses and eating them. This remedy was given to me by a Southern friend, who cannot do without molasses. She learned it from her grandmother.

Raw Onions and Garlic

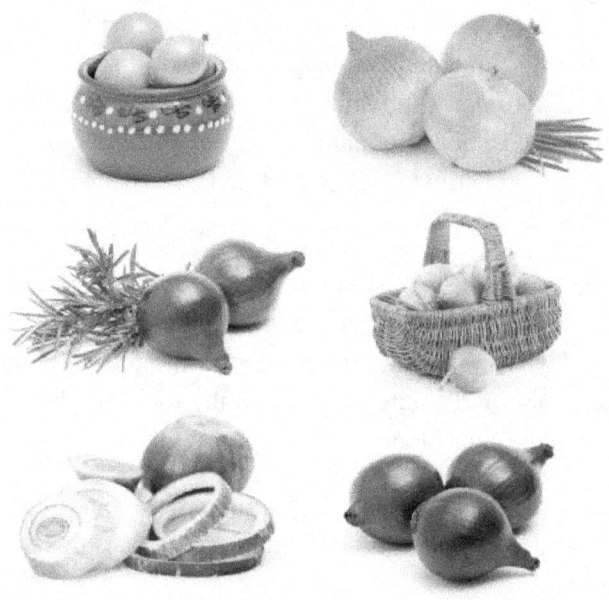

For all those who suffer from constipation, eat one raw onion every meal and stop worrying about your stomach.

Unfortunately, except in Italy and Spain, garlic and raw onion is not an integral part of Western cuisine, which goes by the truthful dictum – An Apple a day keeps the doctor away, but some garlic, a day, keeps everybody away. No wonder, so many people suffer from heart disease. If you can manage to swallow three cloves of raw garlic, every night before sleeping, you would be astonished at the fall of your cholesterol level and a lowering of the possibility of your suffering from heart problems. But no, as the finicky lady in your life gets nauseated by the smell of raw garlic emanating from you, you are not going to eat it. Ah, well.

Garlic is one of the most beneficial of all herbs. An aunt of mine told me this remedy which worked for her. Her piles problem came through not eating fresh fruit and vegetables and suffering from constipation. She mixed 1 teaspoon of fresh mint leaves with a 1 teaspoon of honey and 1 teaspoon lemon juice. She gulped this down 3 times a day for around 15 days and there you are, she was cured. Needless to say, fresh fruit and vegetables are now an integral part of her daily diet.

The idea of Ginger as the curative for skin diseases is that Ginger is a blood purifier. Come summertime, and you may find yourself suffering from boils, pimples or other skin ailments in which your skin is infected. Do not touch them under any circumstances, because that is going to spread the infection. Also, people suffering from constipation may find their skin ailments aggravated. So here is the remedy –

Eat a salad of five – six pieces of chopped Ginger and lemon juice, – sprinkle your favorite salt on it, and season with spices like pepper and chilis, for some extra zing- every day without fail, all through the summer. Not only is it going to be beneficial for your overall state of health in the long run, but also it is going to purify any problems in your blood.

Ancient Greek medicine recommended this ginger and lemon juice mixture as a part of Greek cuisine every day. In fact, I am very pleased to see it in Thai and Chinese kitchens too.

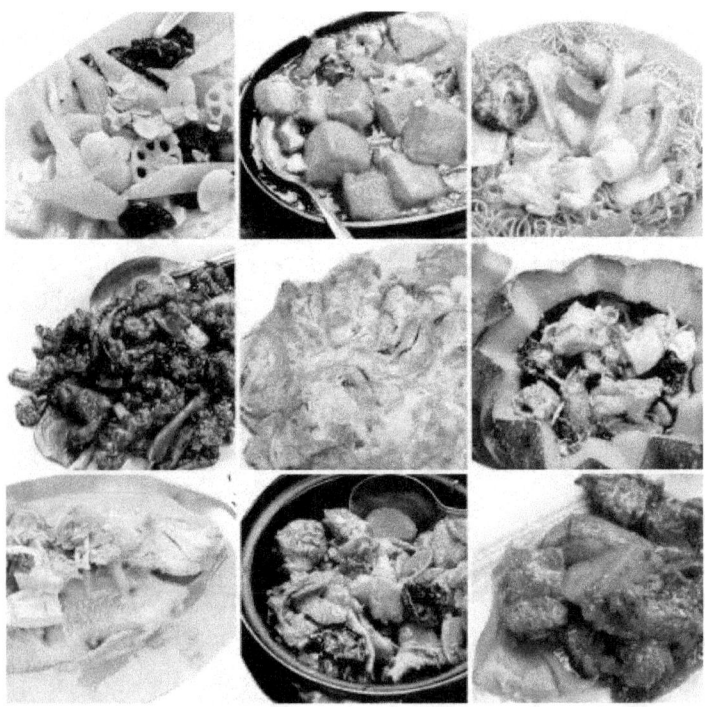

All of these delicious dishes have plenty of ginger in them. Also, you are going to eat Ginger with lemon juice to get rid of the indigestion, which comes from overeating. But what a way to go!

Ginger

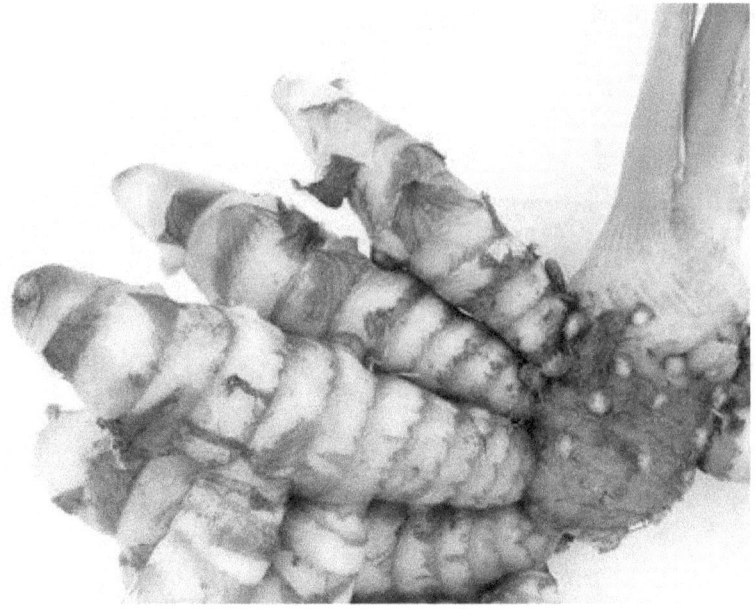

If you are suffering from digestive problems like constipation, gas, and no appetite and the idea of having a meal fills you with fear and trembling, here is a remedy, which I am sure is going to help you.

Chop 5 g of Ginger into small pieces and salt them with your favorite rock salt. This salt is comparatively healthier. Eat them, for 10 days, and voilà, you are going to be eating like a horse.

In the same way, if you have managed to overeat, and you are worried about possible nausea, just allow a piece of ginger to rest a while in your mouth, sucking the juice. This also helps in preventing constipation.

Pomegranates

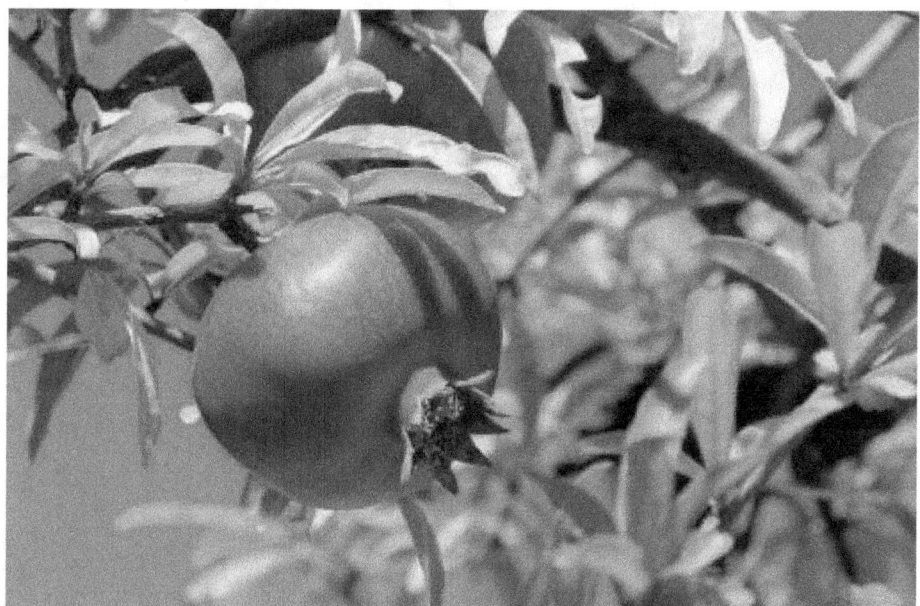

Pomegranate juice has been used in the East, for a long time to get rid of constipation, and also to get your digestive system moving. The pomegranate seed has a mixture of tastes, sweet, sour, a little bit of bitterness and even a tangy flavor.

In Chinese medicine, pomegranates were used by the ancients to get rid of dangerous toxins, and to strengthen the mind, heart, body and soul. The idea of ancient medicine is to put the body in harmony with all the elements in it, and around it. The pomegranate does that for you.

Pomegranate Digestive Chutney

Here is a tasty chutney which you can make especially when you know that all the people at your party are going to overeat on rich and spicy food. Green coriander, mint, black salt, pepper, and pomegranate seeds, in proportions you like along with one clove. Put them all in a blender and grind. Encourage your guests to eat this chutney, so that they do not suffer from nausea, constipation and indigestion brought about by gorging rich and spicy dishes.

Using Copper Utensils

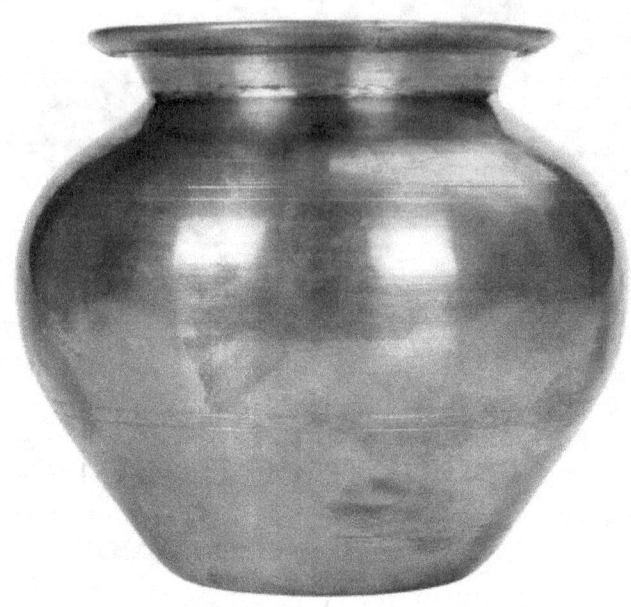

In olden days, you had utensils made out of copper. People stored water in them, and I think that this was a good way in which you could get necessary minerals in your body. So if you have a copper pot anywhere or a copper jug, fill it up with drinking water at night, and drink that water down first thing in the morning.

This prevents constipation and gets your alimentary canal moving. [I tried this out for three days, and I definitely did not suffer from any sort of constipation, running to the bathroom within the next half hour but then I forgot about this way to keep healthy in the daily rush to get ready in order to reach the office in time.]

The problem with constipation is the amount of side effects it has especially feeling lethargic, lazy, pain in the tummy, and a nagging headache. If the constipation is chronic, it can give rise to even more serious ailments. So the first thing to prevent constipation is to eat plenty of fresh fruit and vegetables.

Drink pomegranate juice as often as you can, after eating a spoonful of Bishops Weed.

For people suffering from chronic constipation, this is a remedy, which is been in use for millenniums. You need a copper utensil for this.

These are very common in the East, though they are going out of vogue [or need to come in vogue] in the West. Just place fresh water in a copper utensil, leave it covered throughout the day, and drink it at night. The next morning, you are going to find your system cleared and your constipation gone with the wind, no pun intended. This is the reason why people in the East, do not suffer from chronic constipation. The water utensils placed by the side of their beds are made out of copper, and they drink this water, whenever they wake up during the night.

Flatulence

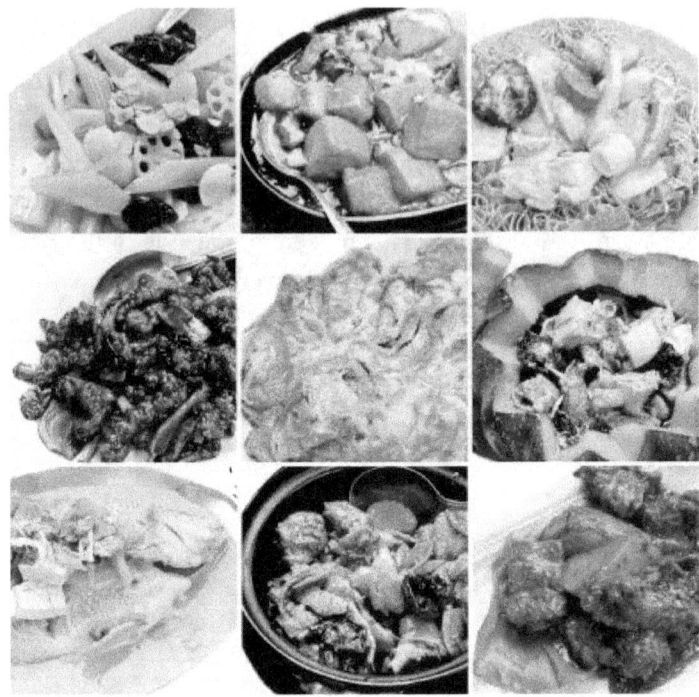

Eating rich indigestible food in summer can give rise to flatulence.

Have you heard of that rather embarrassing word "gas?" This normally occurs when you suffer from constipation, and plenty of toxic gases are produced as a side effect of all that digested food, which is not passing out from your system, thanks to a blocked passage.

Not only can you prevent gas formation in your body, with the use of honey, but also add 5 g honey to 5 g each of ginger and lemon juice, and eat it 3 to 4 times a day to prevent and cure it.

Incidentally, I have found this remedy- honey, ginger and lemon juice- to be an excellent way in which you can manage airsickness and seasickness. It works for me.

In the same way, I manage to get rid of any other digestion related problems by eating half a lemon's juice with a spoonful of honey. Get rid of the worms in your tummy by eating the rind of the lemon.

Flatulence is a rather embarrassing side effect of indigestion and constipation. So if you are suffering from flatulence in the tummy, which can also give rise to headache, nausea, and discomfort in your tummy, try these natural remedies, with the miraculous carrot.

Add 1 teaspoon lemon juice, to one glass carrot juice, with two pinches of soda bicarb. Try drinking this juice mixture, at intervals of two hours, till the flatulence clears up.

Add 1 teaspoon of horseradish juice, four powdered peppercorns and a pinch of asafoetida to half a cup of carrot juice. Asafoetida is the best way in which you can get rid of flatulence and has been used for centuries to cure it.

Heartburn

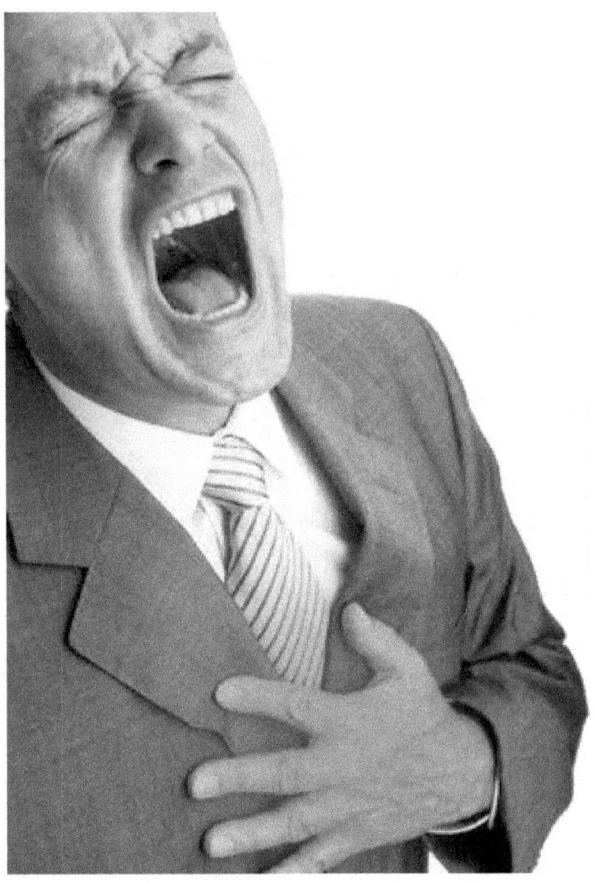

Heartburn, like indigestion Happens When You Eat Heavy and Indigestible Spicy Food

If you are suffering from heartburn, take 5 g each of dried ginger, black pepper, white cumin seeds and small cardamoms. Grind them together and drown them in lemon juice. Dry them for 3 to 4 days in the shade. This dry mixture is very powerful, so whenever you suffer from heartburn, take a pinch of this mixture and swallow with two sips of water. Do this 3 to 4 times a day and get rid/prevent heartburn from ever troubling you again.

If you are suffering from indigestion, all you have to do is mix 1 tablespoon ginger juice with honey and lick the tablespoon clean. Also, before having a heavy meal, drink this digestive – 1 tablespoon lemon and ginger juice with rock salt sprinkled on it. This is going to prevent you from suffering from indigestion. Also, try eating pieces of raw ginger in lemon with your meals. Tasty and good for your digestion.

Piles

Piles is a condition which normally affects people suffering from constipation. Piles is normally a side effect of constipation and many people who eat lots of meat, spicy, fatty and rich foods may find themselves suffering from this problem.

If a patient is suffering from piles, his digestive system is going to go awry. He may not feel hungry, and he may get constipated. He may suffer from flatulence. This affects the digestive system as well as the kidneys, liver and heart adversely. The patient may also have mild facial swelling.

Piles is normally caused by hemorrhoids in the anal region. Sometimes the hemorrhoids burst when a patient is undergoing bowel movements. This causes the passage of blood to be eliminated along with the feces. This is naturally going to cause patients a lot of concern.

Do not eat meat, grapes, and mangoes. When you are suffering from piles, alcohol is forbidden. Eating green leafy vegetables to prevent constipation is advised. Eat 1 tablespoon of honey two times a day to cure piles.

Bloating

Constipation is an extremely common ailment. So the next time you find your stomach bloating, you suffering from flatulence, and you are troubled with indigestion, all you have to do is mix up one and a half teaspoons each of bishops weed, fennel seeds, and black salt with 1 teaspoon of pepper. Powder them together and put them in one glass of water. Drink down. This is going to cure your constipation.

For all those people who have linseed and flaxseeds growing in their gardens, naturally, they are going to be using these seeds and nuts to get their systems moving. But did they know that linseed and flaxseeds leaves can be made into a delicious dish, like any other green leafy vegetable? This is a great flatulence, preventive, while flax is normally used to prevent constipation

Healthy Sprouts Mix

Try this chutney, with your meals. This is extremely healthy, because it is made up of **20 g sprouted mung and 10 g each of sprouted chickpeas and fenugreek.** To this, add **5 g of peanuts seeds and 10 g each of mint and green coriander.**

Then take **5 g each of ginger, Tulsi leaves, molasses, – dates for diabetics – rock salt and garlic.**

Mix them all together and add one days spoonful of lemon juice to it, along with **15 g coconut water.**

This is an extremely delicious chutney, which is rich in potassium, protein, calcium, sulfur, and also really good Digestive enzymes. This is recommended for people suffering from lethargy, acidity, constipation, Also, if you are suffering from stress and strain, this is an excellent tonic to calm you down.

Conclusion

About 50 years ago, many people began to think that the battle against diseases was going to be won decisively with the help of wonder drugs, new, state-of-the-art medical technology and healing methods being used by doctors.

Unfortunately , this has turned out to be a pipe dream, with many of the drugs, giving us more problems than curing the disease. This is in the form of side effects.

One of the main ailments which it has been impossible to wipe out down the ages, like the common cold, is constipation.

This is one of the most common of ailments, brought about through bad dietary habits, and lack of exercise. So the next time you suffer from constipation, do not go in for drugs or for remedies which may be temporary, but which are not going to be effective in the long run.

You need to look for time-tested natural remedies, passed down through centuries, and helping heal and cure millions of people down the ages. These natural cures do not have any side effects. The best thing about them is that they are not results of trial and error serendipity.

This happens to be the prevalent method, which is very common in medical circles today. It can be described on the lines of "if this medicine and treatment does not work, or you, do not worry, we have another medicine coming in in about a week or so. We are going to test it out on you."

Human beings are not guinea pigs. That is why any doctor who has decided that if any medicine fails, he can always get the disease treated with another medicine, is going to be about as lethal to the sake of your well-being as the treatment itself!

So, look at this natural remedies book to cure chronic constipation and take full advantage and benefit of the knowledge of the ages.

Live Long and Prosper!

Author Bio-

Dueep Jyot Singh is a Management and IT Professional who managed to gather Postgraduate qualifications in Management and English and Degrees in Science, French and Education while pursuing different enjoyable career options like being an hospital administrator, IT,SEO and HRD Database Manager/ trainer, movie , radio and TV scriptwriter, theatre artiste and public speaker, lecturer in French, Marketing and Advertising, ex-Editor of Hearts On Fire (now known as Solstice) Books Missouri USA, advice columnist and cartoonist, publisher and Aviation School trainer, ex- moderator on Medico.in, banker, student councilor ,travelogue writer … among other things!

One fine morning, she decided that she had enough of killing herself by Degrees and went back to her first love -- writing. It's more enjoyable! She already has 48 published academic and 14 fiction- in- different- genre books under her belt.

When she is not designing websites or making Graphic design illustrations for clients , she is browsing through old bookshops hunting for treasures, of which she has an enviable collection – including R.L. Stevenson, O.Henry, Dornford Yates, Maurice Walsh, De Maupassant, Victor Hugo, Sapper, C.N. Williamson, "Bartimeus" and the crown of her collection- Dickens "The Old Curiosity Shop," and so on… Just call her "Renaissance Woman") - collecting herbal remedies, acting like Universal Helping Hand/Agony Aunt, or escaping to her dear mountains for a bit of exploring, collecting herbs and plants and trekking.

Our books are available at

1. Amazon.com
2. Barnes and Noble
3. Itunes
4. Kobo
5. Smashwords
6. Google Play Books

Check out some of the other JD-Biz Publishing books
Gardening Series on Amazon

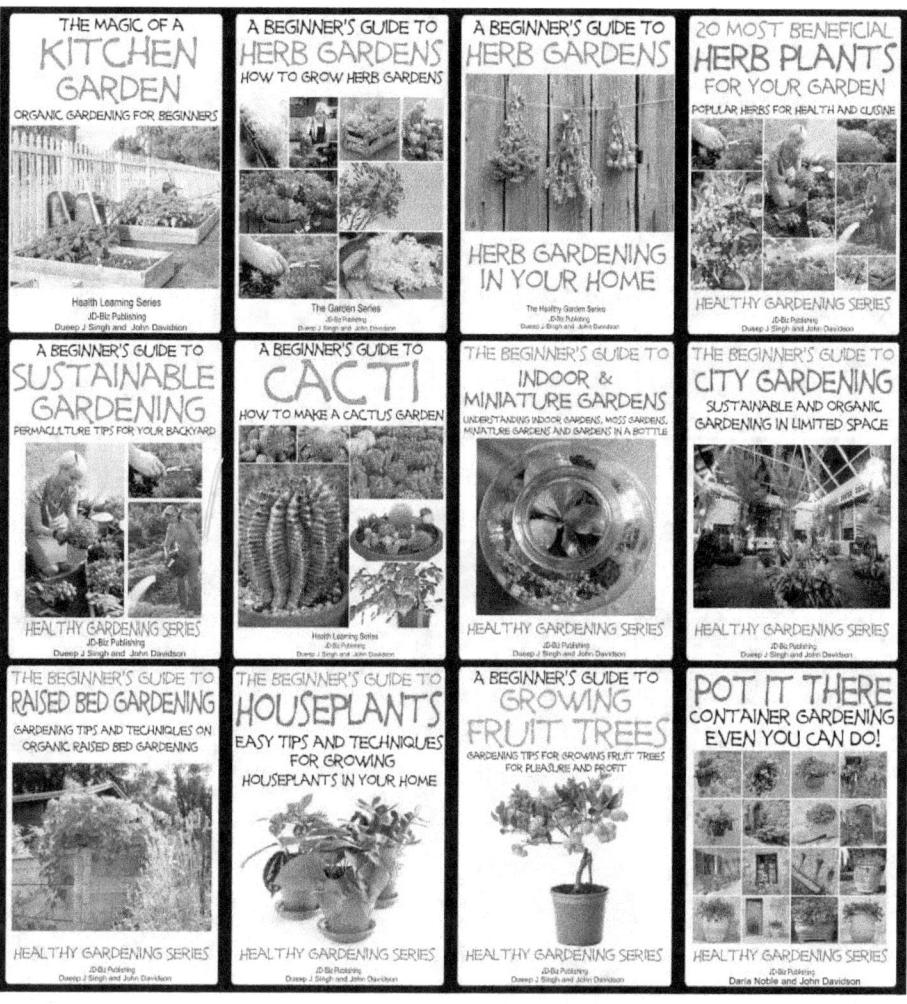

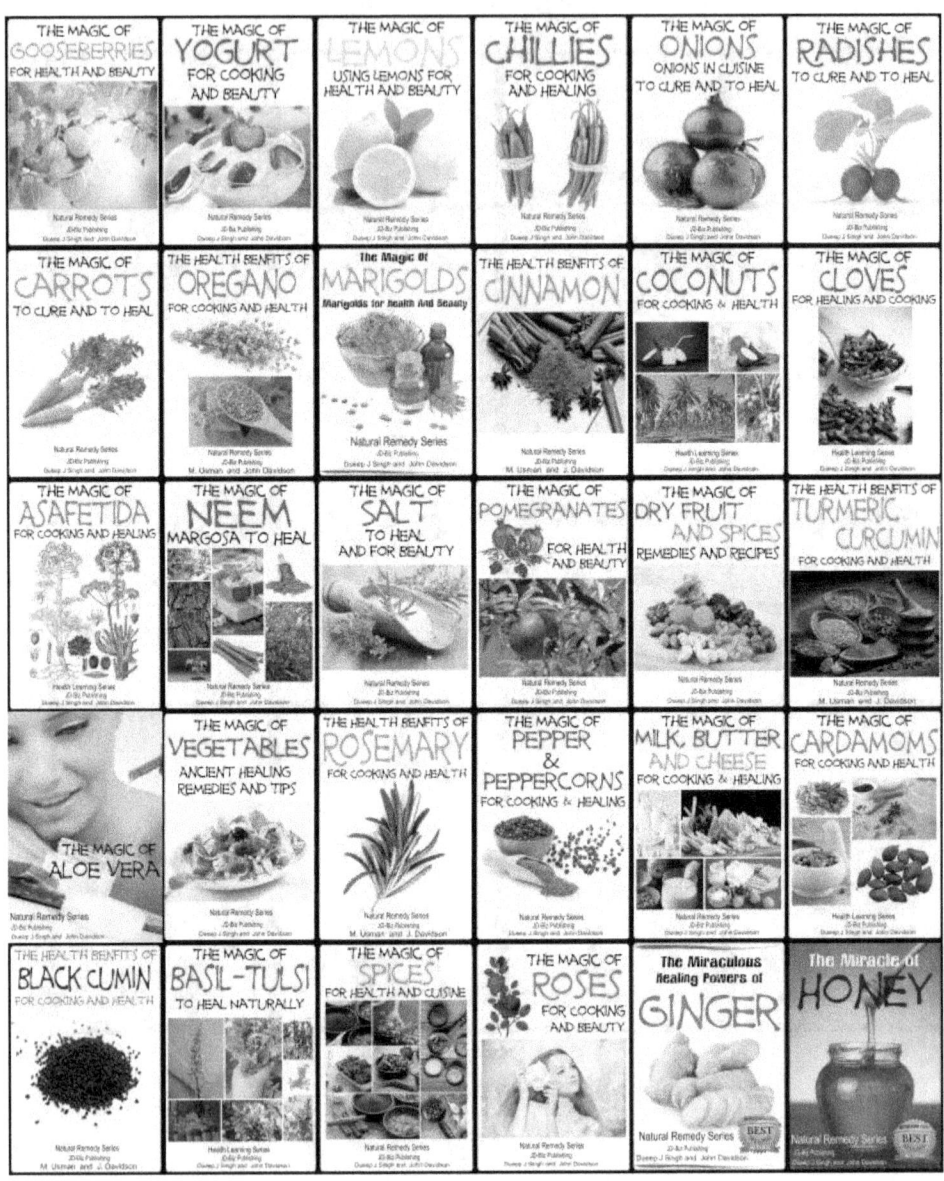

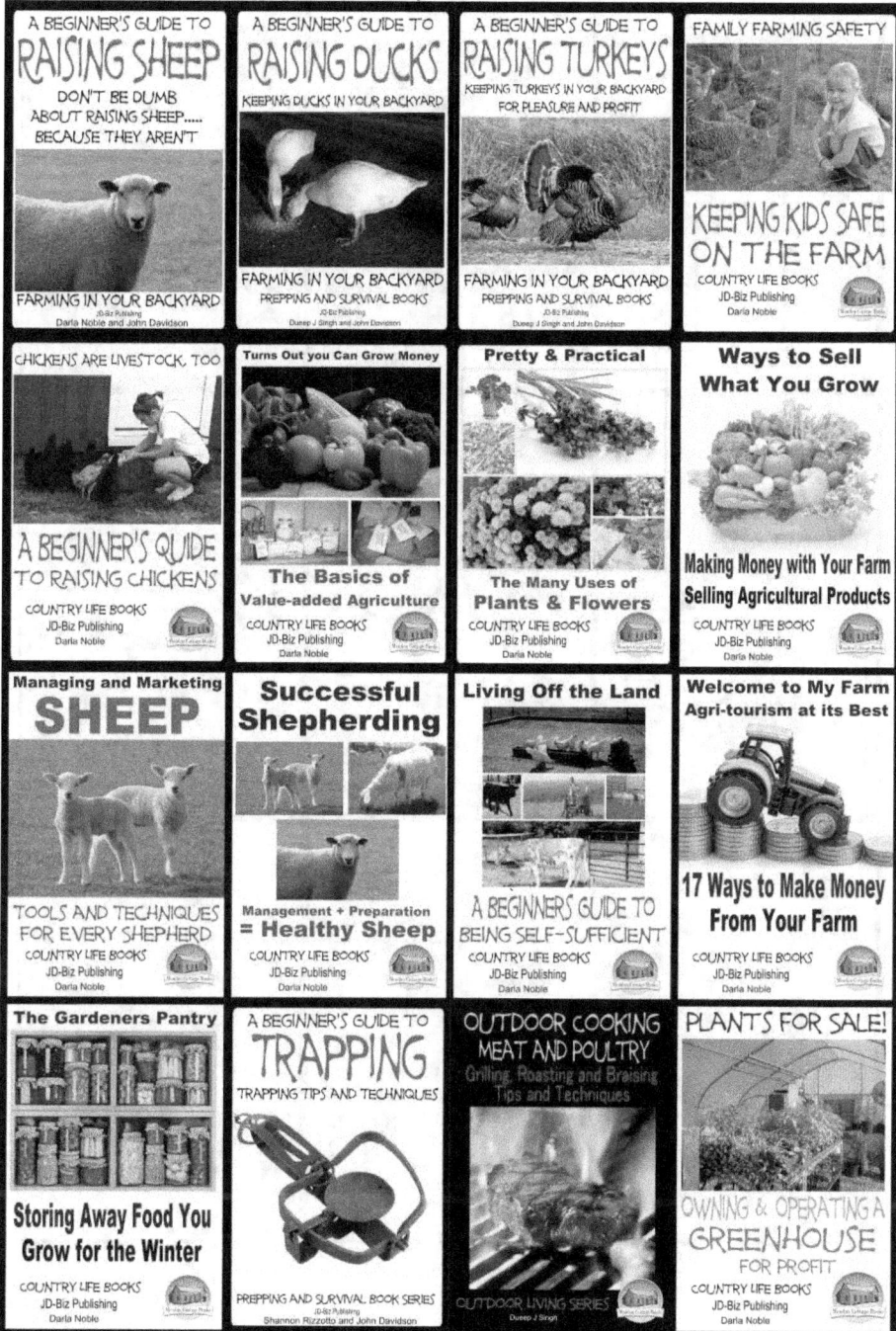

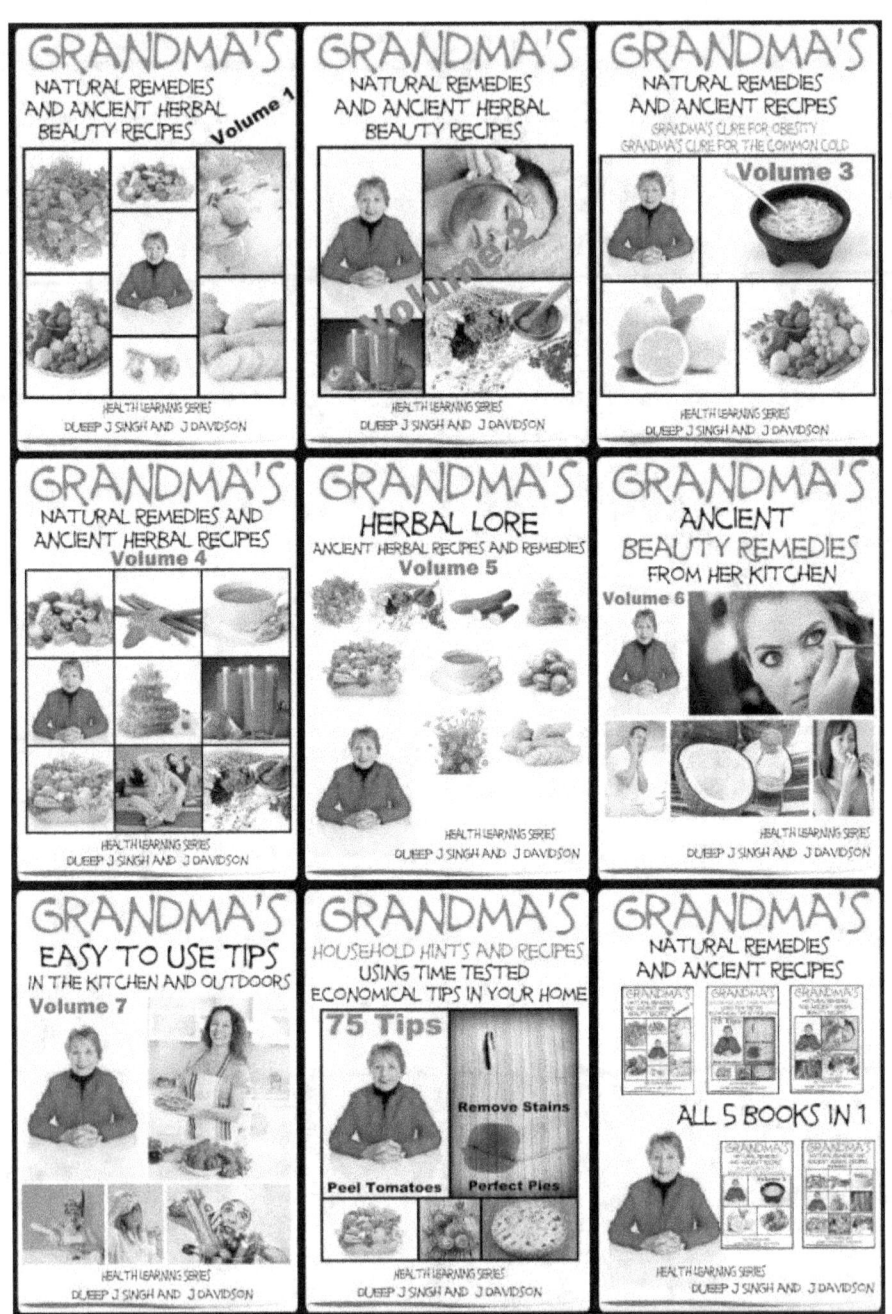

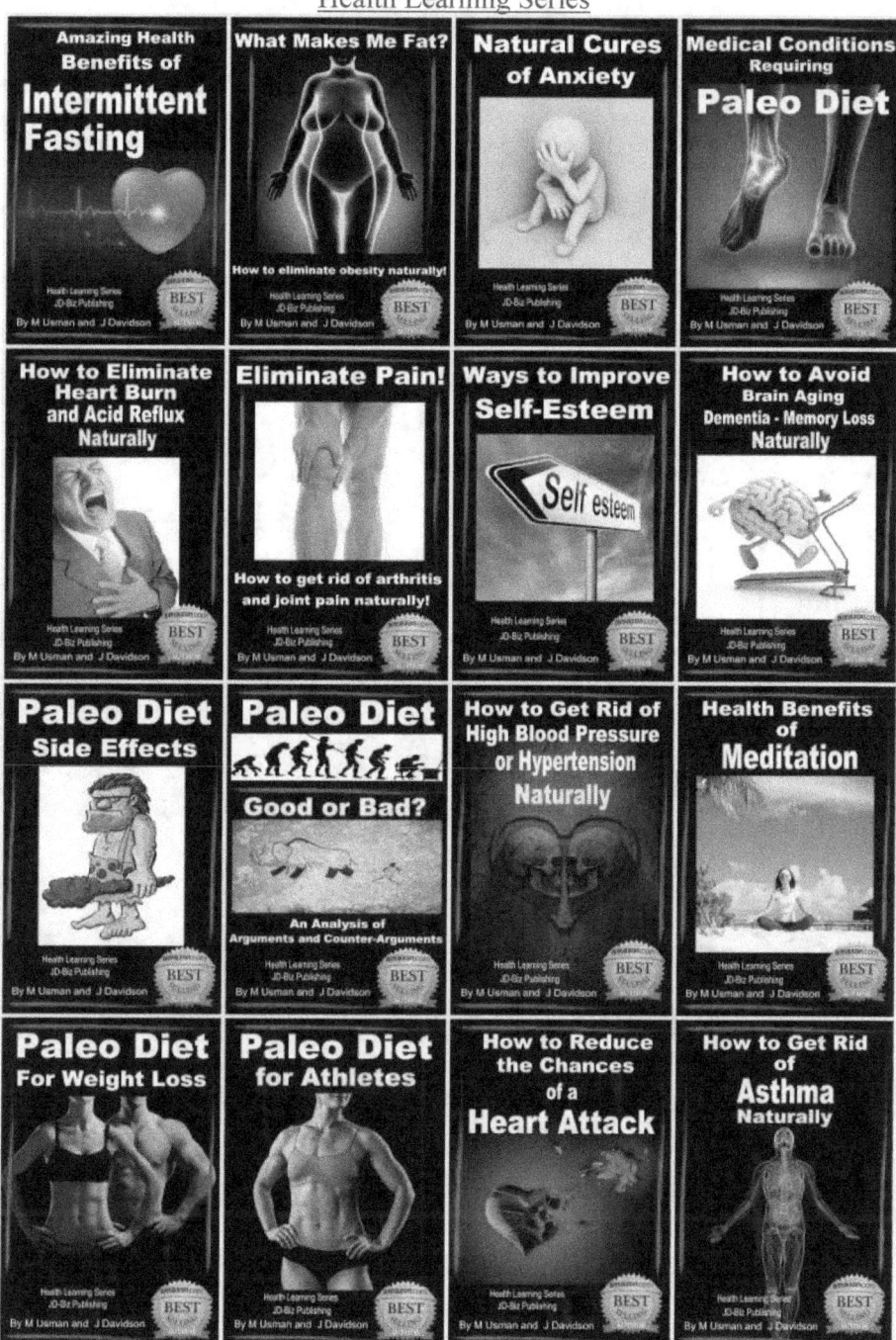

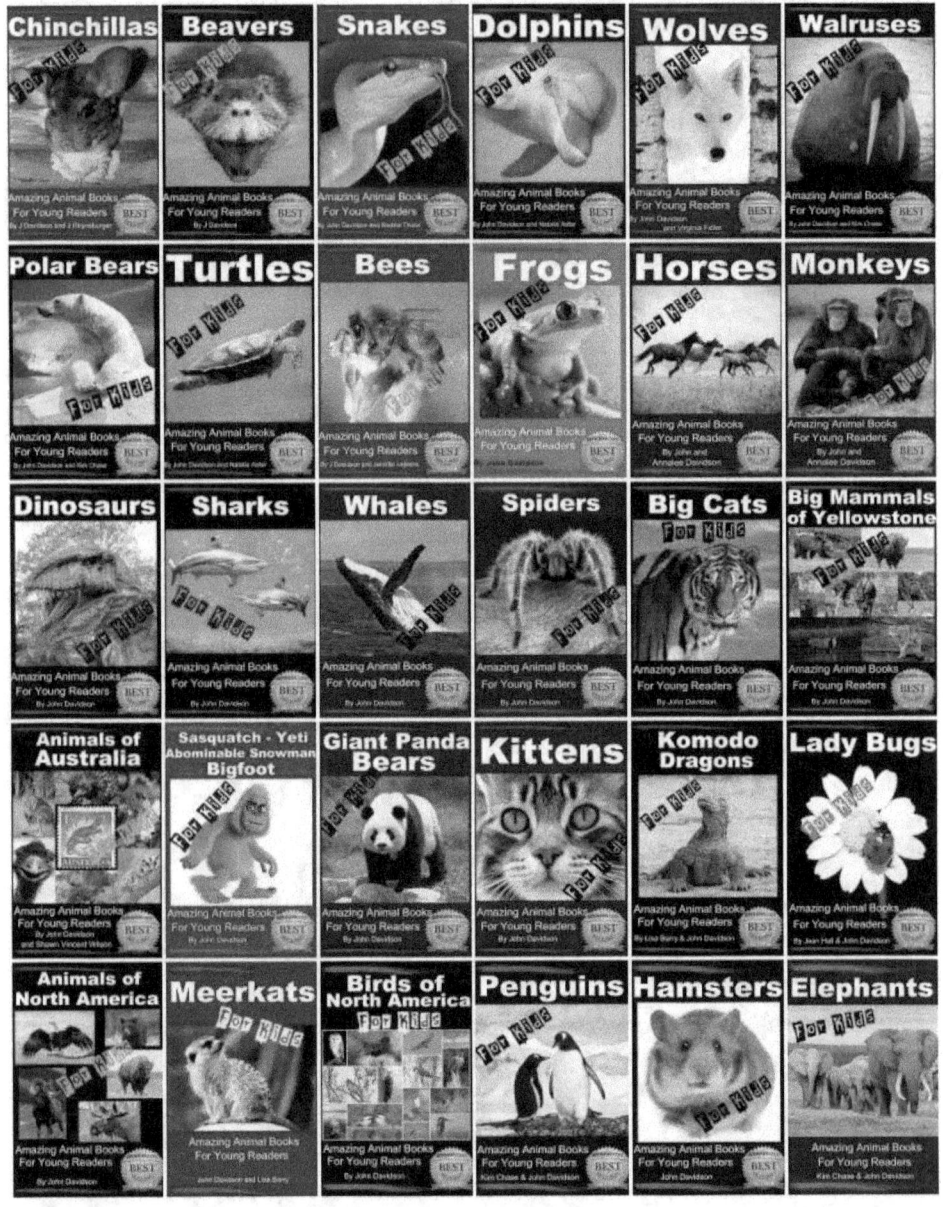

Learn To Draw Series

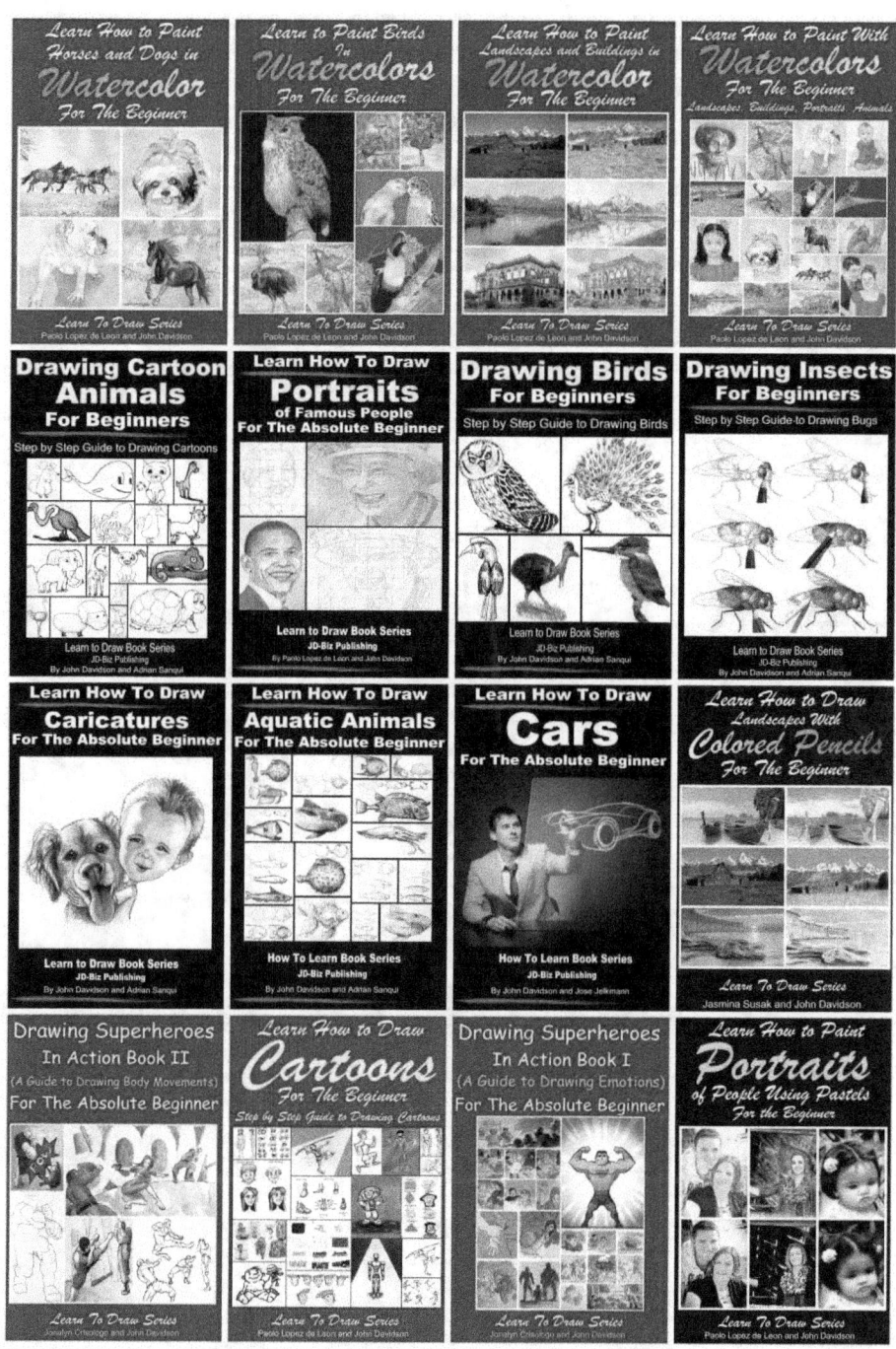

How to Build and Plan Books

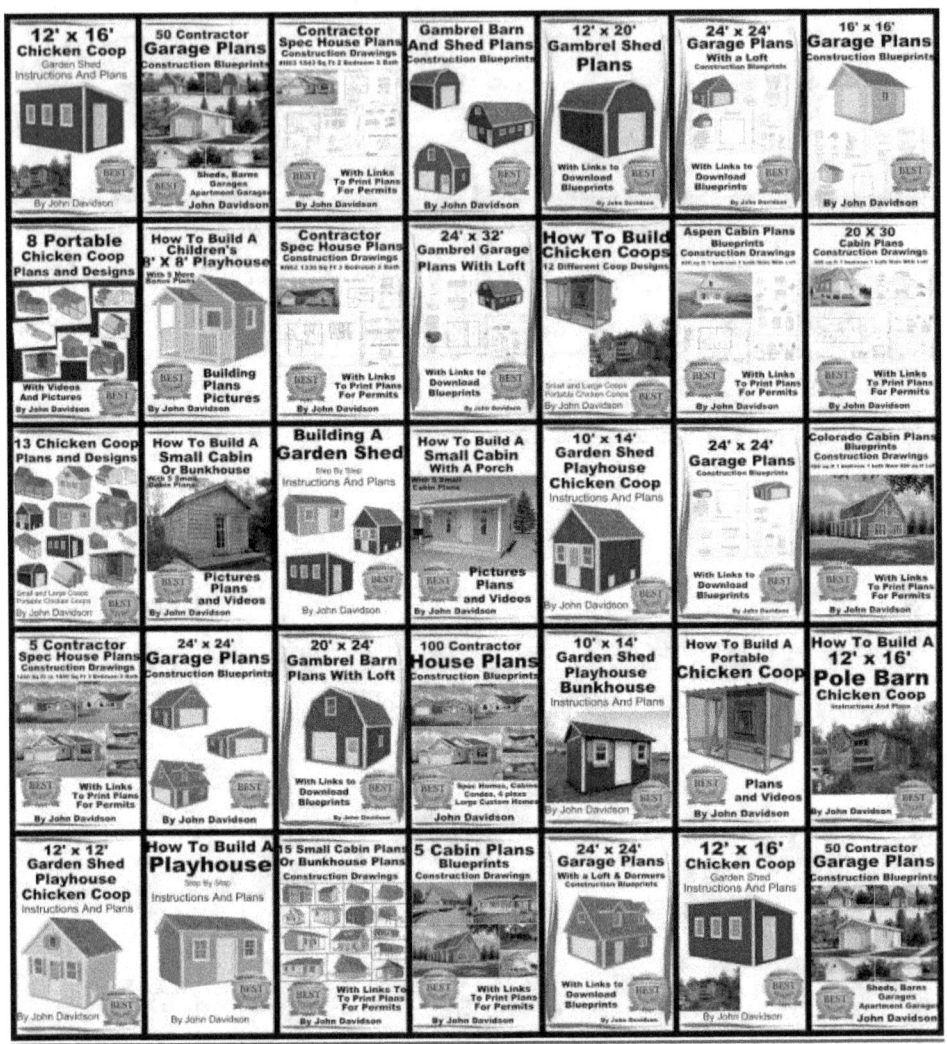

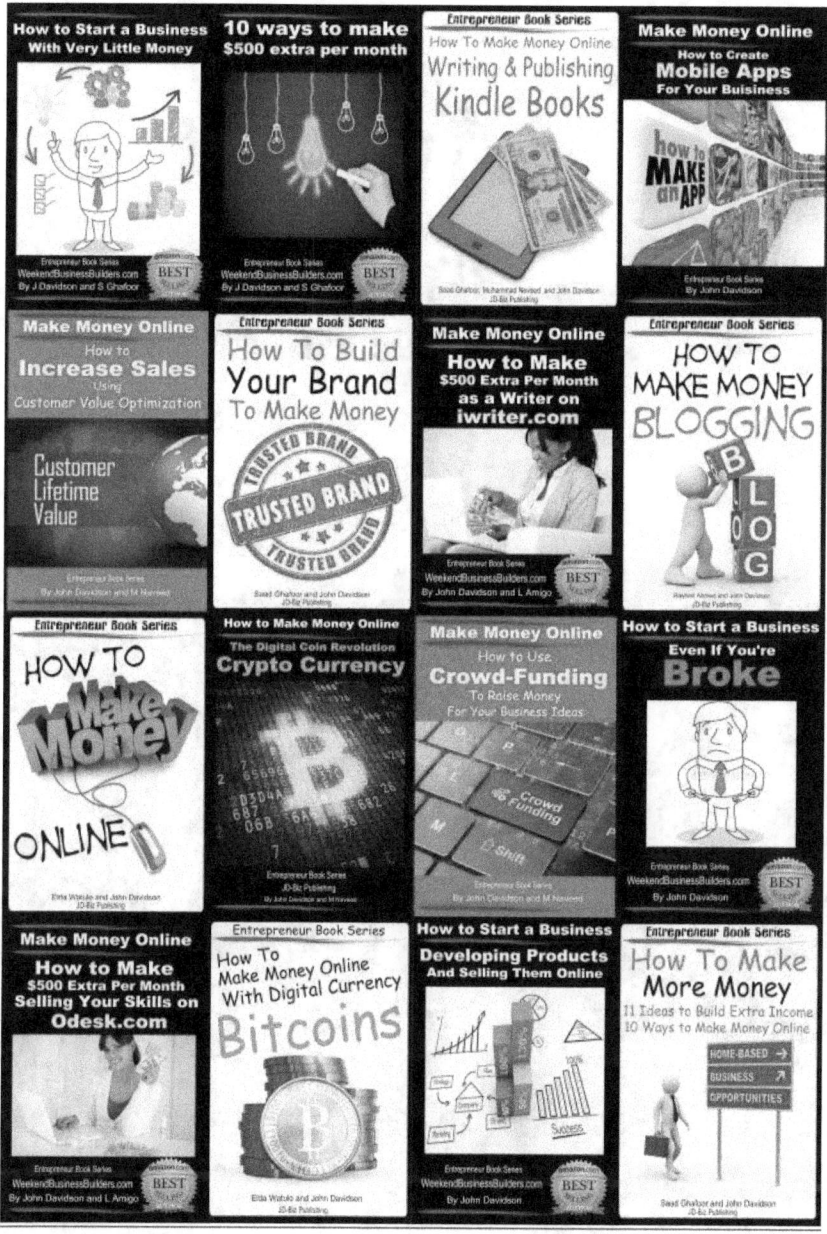

Publisher

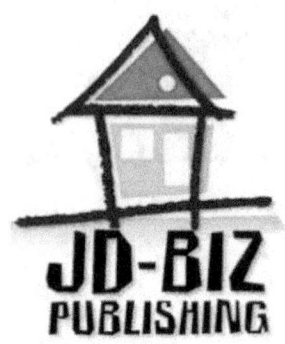

JD-Biz Corp

P O Box 374

Mendon, Utah 84325

http://www.jd-biz.com/

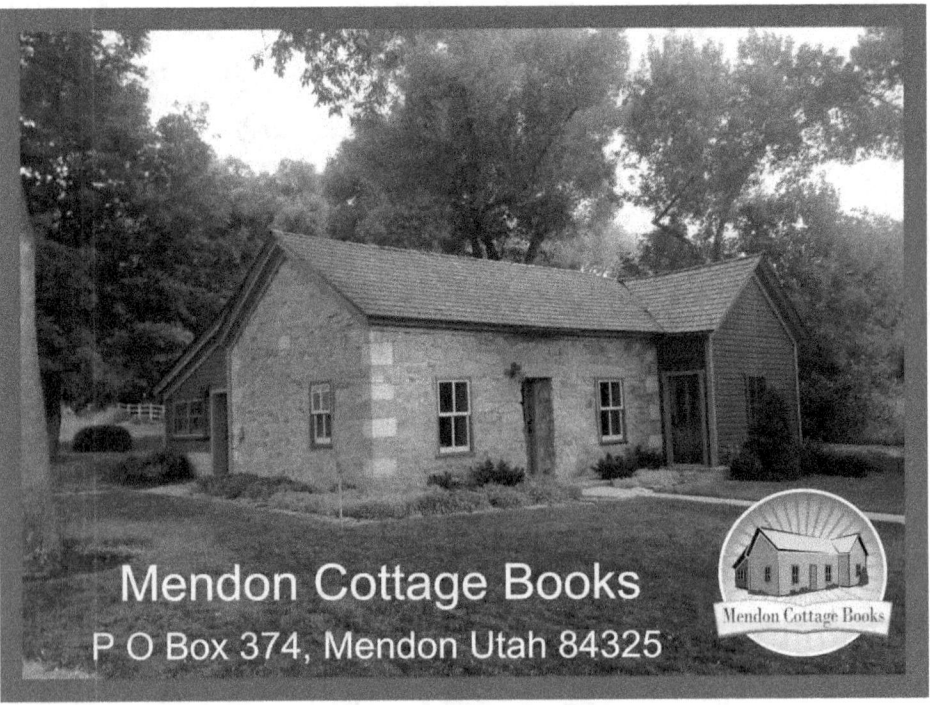

Mendon Cottage Books

P O Box 374, Mendon Utah 84325

www.ingramcontent.com/pod-product-compliance
Lightning Source LLC
Chambersburg PA
CBHW072017290526
45787CB00013B/1286